USMLE STEP 2 CK
Dermatology
In Your Pocket

✓ Study guide for the USMLE STEP 2 CK exam.

✓ Prepare for your shelf examination.

✓ Be ready for your inpatient rotation.

Gregory J. Fernandez, M.D.

This book is gratefully dedicated to my wife. Thank you for your support and always being there for me. Thank you for your kindness, your devotion, and your endless selflessness support. I love you... Thank you mother, father, step-mother, brothers, friends, and family for all your encouragement and endless love. Best of luck to all the medical dreamers, the road is long and I hope my book helps you through this journey. All the best...

First Edition, 2016

Author & Editor: Gregory J. Fernandez, M.D.

Publisher: M.D. Educational Services

Book Design: Marie Meyer

Copyediting: Editage Cactus Communications

ISBN-13: 978-1530285662

ISBN-10: 1530285666

How to Use

"Dermatology In Your Pocket"

Dermatology In Your Pocket is a study guide for the USMLE STEP 2 CK exam that you can also use to prepare for your shelf examination and to get ready for your inpatient rotation. It is part of a series, each dealing with a different subject or sub-specialty, focusing on vital clinical knowledge.

The subjects and topics within dermatology are called out in large, colored type. These items are also included in the Table of Contents for ease of access.

Many subjects also contain sub-subjects that are also called out in bold, blue type either as bulleted items or in-line with the text, as appropriate. They are all referenced in the index.

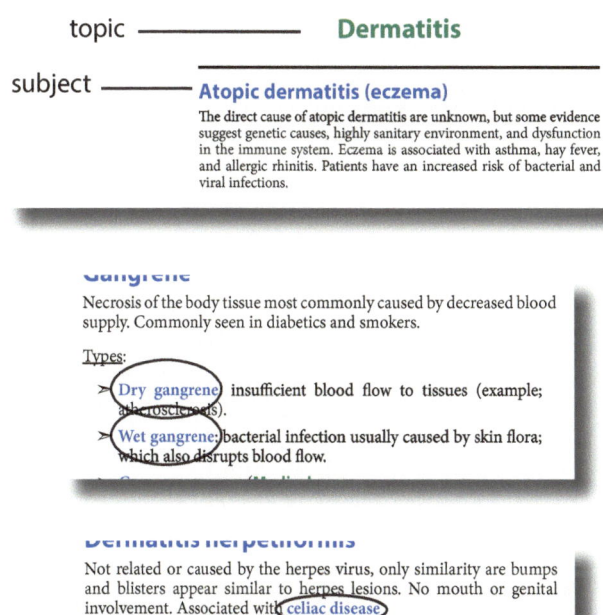

Presentation of clinical history and physical exam (Hx/PE), step-by-step diagnosis, and treatment plan are indicated by bold red headings.

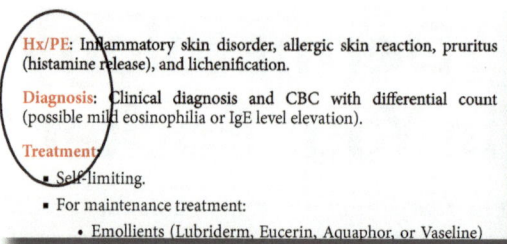

Procedures, triads, pathology, medications, antibodies and findings are called out in bold text. These items are also included in the index.

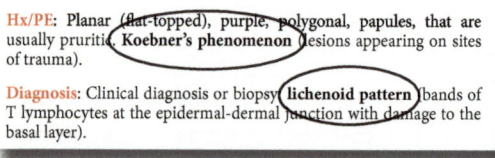

Reflexes, signs and maneuvers are shown in purple text.

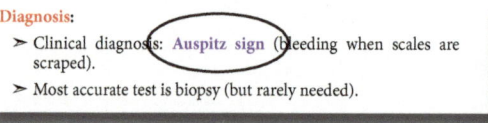

Mnemonics and key words are shown in orange text.

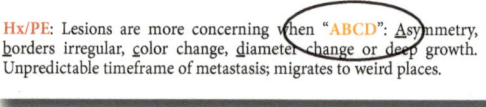

And, finally, for the avoidance of doubt, circumstances that amount to a medical emergency are flagged with warning.

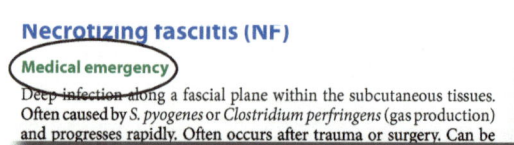

Dermatology
Table of Contents

Dermatitis

Atopic dermatitis (eczema)

The direct cause of atopic dermatitis are unknown, but some evidence suggest genetic causes, highly sanitary environment, and dysfunction in the immune system. Eczema is associated with asthma, hay fever, and allergic rhinitis. Patients have an increased risk of bacterial and viral infections.

<u>Triggers</u>: food, climate, contact allergens, chemicals, topical antibiotics, and emotional disturbance.

Hx/PE: Inflammatory skin disorder, allergic skin reaction, pruritus (histamine release), and lichenification.

Diagnosis: Clinical diagnosis and CBC with differential count (possible mild eosinophilia or IgE level elevation).

Treatment:

- Self-limiting and avoidance of triggers
- For maintenance treatment:
  - Best long-term therapy: emollients (Lubriderm, Eucerin, Aquaphor, or Vaseline) for skin hydration (best long-term therapy).
  - Low-potency topical glucocorticoids can be used for longer periods of time compared to topical high dose steroids.
- In case of *severe* flare-up, use higher-potency topical steroids.
  - Higher-potency steroids are not usually recommended for more than 2 weeks.
- Anti-histamines for treatment of pruritus.

<u>Prevention</u>: use prophylactic non-drying soaps, non-scented moisturizers, and avoid triggers. Avoid oral steroids owing to their side effects unless absolutely needed.

Contact dermatitis

A type IV hypersensitivity reaction (T-cells), which is trigged by contact with an allergen or irritant. Patients with previous exposure and now re-exposed to the allergen or irritant.

Triggers: poison ivy, poison oak, nickel (*most common* metal), latex, rubber, PPD, and cosmetics.

Types:

➤ Acute: erythema and thin blisters followed by scaling and crusting.

➤ Chronic: erythema and lichenification.

Hx/PE: Mild fever, localized edema, pruritus, rash (often thin blisters), and lymphadenopathy. The rash usually mimics the pattern of the allergy-causing the reaction.

Diagnosis: Clinical diagnosis and if unsure perform **patch test** (an allergen test that can be helpful to identify the allergen).

Treatment:

- *Mild or moderate cases*, avoid triggers and use low dose topical steroids and wet cold compressions.

- Severe cases or not respond to low-dose steroids, then use high-dose topical steroids or systemic corticosteroids.

- Poison oak: treat with topical corticosteroids, cold compression, and oatmeal application.

Prophylaxis: avoid triggers (most important) and use non-drying/non-scented soaps and moisturizers.

Hypersensitivity reactions

Types of hypersensitivity reactions: "ACID" anaphylactic, cytotoxic, immune complex, and delayed.

Type I (anaphylactic)

An anaphylactic reaction, which cuases a release of IgE, mast cells, basophils, and histamines. Local wheal and flares. Associated with asthma and allergies.

Type II (cytotoxic)

An immune response that releases IgM and IgG antibodies that bind to the antigens on the enemy cells and cause lysis via complement products. Involves the activation of the membrane attack complex (MAC).

Type III (immune complex)

Antigen–antibody complexes activate the complement products that attract neutrophils and release lysosomal enzymes.

Subtypes:

➤ **Serum sickness**: commonly caused by medications; occurs about a week after exposure.

➤ **Arthus reaction**: antibody-mediated hypersensitivity reaction; occurs after intradermal injection of an antigen. Causes an antigen-antibody complex reaction in the skin.

Type IV delayed (cell mediated)

Cell mediated T lymphocytes encounter the antigens, which leads to macrophage activation.

Risk factors: PPD skin test, contact dermatitis, poison ivy, and poison oak.

Erythema nodosum (EN)

An inflammatory process probably related to a type IV hypersensitivity reaction to a variety of antigens. Patients present with **panniculitis** (inflamed fat cells under skin) usually over the tibia.

<u>Triggered by</u>: infections, drug reactions (sulfas and OCPs), chronic inflammatory disease (ulcerative colitis and Crohn's disease), histoplasmosis, sarcoidosis, coccidioidomycosis, and tuberculosis.

Hx/PE: <u>Painful</u> pretibial tenderness. Lesions are reddish-brown subcutaneous nodules, usually found in the lower extremities.

Diagnosis:

- Clinical diagnosis or biopsy (histological [septal panniculitis]).
- <u>Additional evaluation considerations</u>:
    - Post-streptococcal glomerulonephritis: ASO titer.
    - Infection or cellulitis: ESR.
    - Tuberculosis: PPD.
    - Inflammatory bowel disease: small bowel series.
    - Sarcoidosis, coccidioidomycosis, and histoplasmosis: chest radiography.

Treatment:

- Self-limiting within 3-6 weeks.
- Leg elevation, rest, compressive bandages.
- NSAIDs and analgesics. NSAIDs can be helpful for pain but chronic use may lead to erythema multiforme (EM).

Pityriasis rosea

Acute dermatitis where lesions are pink and scaly (salmon colored). Possible association with herpes virus (HHV-6 or HHV-7).

Hx/PE:

- <u>Initial lesion</u>: "**herald patch**."
- <u>Secondary lesion</u>: "**cigarette paper**" and classic "**Christmas tree**" patterns.
    - Erythema with peripheral scales. Never involves the palms or soles.

Diagnosis: Clinical diagnosis or can use KOH (rule out fungal infection) and VDRL (rule out syphilis).

Treatment:

- Self-limiting (weeks to months).
- Use non-drying lotions and anti-pruritics (anti-histamine).
- Severe cases: short-term topical steroids, which are more used to decrease pruritus.
- Acyclovir may decrease the duration and severity.

Acanthosis nigricans

Hyperpigmentation in the intertriginous zones (neck, axilla, and groin). Associated with GI malignancy and other conditions related to insulin resistance such as Cushing's syndrome and PCOS.

Hx/PE: Hyperkeratotic lesions with a "velvety appearance."

Diagnosis:

- Clinical diagnosis.
- Rule out diabetes, Cushing's syndrome, PCOS, steroid use, and obesity.

Treatment:

- Control underlying causes; for example, lose weight and control diabetes.
- Topical retinoids can be helpful.

Lichen planus

The cause is unknown but thought to be an autoimmune process. Causes chronic inflammatory dermatosis (inflammation of the skin) and/or mucous membrane involvement. Associated with advanced HCV infection.

Hx/PE: Planar (flat-topped), purple, polygonal, papules, that are usually pruritic. **Koebner's phenomenon** (lesions appearing on sites of trauma).

Diagnosis: Clinical diagnosis or biopsy: **lichenoid pattern** (bands of T lymphocytes at the epidermal-dermal junction with damage to the basal layer).

Treatment:

- No cure and usually resolves spontaneously in about 6 months for cutaneous lesions and longer for mucosal lesion.
- Topical steroids and tretinoin may be helpful.

Rosacea

A chronic skin condition of redness and dilated blood vessels of the face. The direct cause is unknown but studies show an increase in *demodex* mites numbers on skin. Rosacea is associated with **rhinophyma** (prominent pores and a fibrous thickening of the nose) and ocular keratitis (the cornea becomes inflamed).

Hx/PE: Patients tend to have abnormal flushing response to various substances such as heat, cold, food, and emotional disturbance.

➤ Early: central facial erythema.

➤ Later: papules and pustules.

Diagnosis: Clinical diagnosis and need to rule out SLE "**butterfly rash pattern**)".

Treatment:

- Avoid triggers such as heat, cold, foods, and the sun.
- Medications include ivermectin, doxycycline, and isotretinoin.
- Less evidence with topical metronidazole.

Note: Always warn against alcohol use with metronidazole.

Chloasma (melasma)

An abnormally high stimulation of melanocytes that create melanin. Disorder of pigmentation that can effect anyone but are more commonly seen in women who are pregnancy or taking OCPs.

Diagnosis: Clinical diagnosis (irregular hyperpigmented macules or patches) or **wood lamp** (increased melanin).

Treatment: Discontinue OCPs, topical hydroquinone 4% (bleaching creams), topical tretinoin, sunscreen, and avoiding direct sun exposure.

Urticaria

Urticaria (hives)

Severity can range from itchy bumps to life-threatening anaphylaxis. Lesions are usually acute with superficial with localized edema, usually acute but can be chronic. Reaction is similar to type I hypersensitivity reaction where there is a release of IgE, histamine, basophiles, prostaglandins, and mast cells.

Severe cases: tongue swelling, angioedema, asthma, and fever.

Hx/PE: Lesions with pruritus, erythematous plaques, and raised-skin lesions (wheals or welts) of various sizes. Lesions can appear as a pale halo edematous centralized lesion surrounded by an erythematous area. Usually last up to 24 hours and fade away.

Diagnosis:

- Clinical diagnosis or can also confirmation with biopsy (shows perivascular edema).
- **Allergy test** might give insight on allergen.

Treatment:

- *First step* is to avoid triggers.
- *First line medications* are systemic anti-histamines.
- Systemic steroids can be used in extreme cases.
- Topical medications offer no benefit here.

Drug-induced dermatology

Fixed drug eruption

Usually observed about 7–14 days after treatment with a new drug. If a rash develops a few days after starting a drug, it is probably not the cause. All four types of hypersensitivity reactions are possible with fixed drug eruption.

<u>Risk</u> of developing Stevens Johnson's syndrome (SJS) or toxic epidermal necrosis (TEN).

Hx/PE: Patients usually present with a pruritic relatively symmetrical reddish macules or papules in the same area. After the condition resolves, patients often present with persistent brown pigmentation.

Diagnosis: Clinical diagnosis (patient on new medication) or CBC with differentials (may show eosinophilia).

Treatment: Stop the medication and administer anti-histamines (helps pruritus).

Neurodermatitis

Lichen simplex chronicus (LSC)

A skin condition caused be chronic rubbing or scratching.

Hx/PE: Lichenified, excoriated, and hyperpigmented plaques.

Diagnosis: Clinical diagnosis that maybe associated with depression, anxiety, or nervousness.

Treatment: Mild topical steroids and oral anti-histamines (for pruritus).

Autoimmune dermatitis

Pemphigus vulgaris

Autoimmune disease against **desmoglein**, which attaches and joins epidermal cells to desmosomes. The disease causes intra-epidermal blisters leading to widespread painful erosions of the skin and mucosa.

Hx/PE: Usually causes mucous ulcers, which can progress to skin involvement. Rarely intact blister because of erosion of the epidermis.

Can be very painful but <u>rarely</u> pruritic.

Diagnosis:

- Clinical diagnosis (<u>positive</u> Nikolsky's sign).
- *Most accurate test*: skin biopsy with direct immunofluorescence or ELISA test (**anti-desmoglein antibodies**).

Treatment: Initially, <u>systemic</u> corticosteroids at a high dose, followed by azathioprine and IVIG.

Bullous pemphigoid

Autoimmune disease in elderly patients (70s and 80s); rare in children, with less mucus involvement and deeper separation at the epidermal basement membrane junction.

Hx/PE: Firm and stable blisters (<u>negative</u> Nikolsky's sign).

Diagnosis:

- Clinical diagnosis or biopsy from the edge of blister for confirmation (subepidermal blisters often with abundant eosinophils).
  - Requires two skin biopsies: one for **H&E staining** and one for immunofluorescence testing.
    - Linear IgG and C3 immunoglobulins and complement at the dermal-epidermal junction.

Treatment:

- *Mild localized disease*: topical corticosteroids appears as effective as systemic.
- *Severe wide spread disease:* systemic steroids followed by azathioprine.

Vitiligo

A chronic progressive autoimmune depigmentation disease of the skin. Most common in the dorsal hands, periorificial face, and genitalia. Associated with other autoimmune disorders, commonly Hashimoto's, DMI, and Grave's disease.

Hx/PE: Sharply demarcated pigmented macules or patches.

Diagnosis:

- Clinical diagnosis.
- **Ultraviolet light** (black light) lesion appear blue.
- If needed, skin biopsy (total absence of melanocytes).

Treatment:

- Topical steroids and phototherapy.
- Topical or systemic psoralens, exposure to sunlight, or PUVA (psoralens + UVA).
- Apply sunscreen, dyes, and make-up may be helpful.

Note: A patient with malignant melanoma can develop an **anti-melanocyte** immune response that leads to vitiligo.

Keloids

A benign overgrowth of granulation tissue, fibrotic tissue, and collagen type I tissue leading to the formation of scar tissue that extends beyond the border of the original wound. More common in those of African descent.

Diagnosis: Clinical diagnosis.

Treatment:

- *Best treatment* is avoidance of trauma and injury.
- *Best medication is* intralesional corticosteroid injection (Kenalog).

Psoriasis

The exact cause of psoriasis is not fully understood but it seems to be associated with an immune-mediated skin disorder, particularly T-cell-mediated inflammatory response. Relapse and remitting is common and disease first becomes apparent in young adults.

Hx/PE: Classically found on extensor surfaces (elbows and knees).

Sharply bordered erythematous patches and "silvery scales on red base."

➤ Psoriatic arthritis: develops only in 5% of the patients with psoriasis. Begins in the hands with "sausage digits" but later involves many joints. In cases of spinal involvement, usually the patient is positive for HLA B-27. However, there is no specific test for psoriatic arthritis.

➤ Onycholysis (psoriatic nails): visual pitting of nail and lifting of nail beds. Seen in psoriatic arthritis.

➤ Pustular psoriasis: can be life threatening (electrolyte abnormalities and loss of serum proteins).

➤ Koebner's phenomenon: provoked by local irritation or trauma.

Diagnosis:

➤ Clinical diagnosis: Auspitz sign (bleeding when scales are scraped).

➤ *Most accurate test* is biopsy (but rarely needed).

  • Munro's microabscess: thick epidermis and absence of granular cells with preservation of nuclei in the stratum corneum.

Treatment:

  ▪ As a rule of thumb: *mild disease* (topical agents), *moderate disease* (phototherapy), and *severe disease* (systemic treatment). There is a wide variety of treatments and will only list a few.

    • Mild or localized disease: topical steroids.

    • Heaped-up lesions: salicylic acid.

    • Widespread disease (>30% of the body): phototherapy including PUVA.

    • Severe disease: combination of methotrexate (MTX), phototherapy, and topical steroids.

    • Psoriatic arthritis: MTX

Prevention: keeping the affected area moist with Eucerin, Lubriderm, Aquaphor, or petroleum jelly (helps with pain and itching).

Note:

✓ MTX can cause liver toxicity (liver fibrosis) and megaloblastic anemia. Take with folic acid supplementation.

✓ β-blockers and lithium can exacerbate psoriatic lesions.

Dermatitis herpetiformis

Not related or caused by the herpes virus, only similarity are bumps and blisters appear similar to herpes lesions. No mouth or genital involvement. Associated with celiac disease.

Hx/PE: Lesions appear similar to herpes virus but do not involve genitals or mouth. Very often overlooked as a diagnosis.

Diagnosis: Blood test (IgA antibodies) and skin biopsy (characterized by papillary dermal neutrophil collections and IgA complex).

Treatment: Gluten-free diet (*most important*) and Dapsone.

Dermatological viral infections

Herpes simplex virus (HSV)

Painful recurrent vesicular eruptions: HSV-1 (oral herpes) and HSV-2 (genital herpes). The epidermal cells fuse into giant cells. Can be transmitted by direct contact and primary episodes are generally longer and more severe. Become dormant in local nerve ganglia. Recurrence limited to the mucocutaneous zone innervated by the involved nerve.

Risk factors: stress, fever, immunosuppression, and sun.

Hx/PE: First presents with skin tingling and burning pain. On physical examination, lesions are referred to as "clustered vesicles on an erythematous base." .

Diagnosis:

- Clinical diagnosis (no other tests usually needed).
- If unsure use Tzanck test (cheap) or *most accurate test* is PCR testing.

Treatment:

- If recurrent herpes or underling HIV, use acyclovir (7–10 days).

- If >6 outbreaks per year: acyclovir daily (prophylaxis).
  - Acyclovir decreases the severity and frequency.
- In cases of infection with resistant herpes, treat with foscarnet.

Note:

- ✓ Condoms are only effective if they cover the infected area. A condom would <u>not</u> be effective if the eruption is in the pubic area or areas not covered
- ✓ Isolation should be ensured for all patients with **disseminated herpes zoster**.
- ✓ Increase H_2O intake while taking acyclovir to avoid ATN.

Behcet's syndrome

Observed in patients with a <u>triad</u> of oral ulcers, genital ulcers, and uveitis. Risk of developing erythema multiforme and involvement of a variety of visceral organs.

Diagnosis: Clinical diagnosis (signs and symptoms) no specific testing.

Treatment:

- <u>Mild cases</u>: topical steroids (genital ulcers), special mouth rinse with steroids (mouth ulcers), and eye drops with steroids (uveitis).

- <u>Moderate to severe</u> cases or immunosuppressed patients: corticosteroids (decrease inflammation) followed by azathioprine.

Varicella-Zoster virus (VZV)

Transferred via respiratory droplet or direct contact. Contagious 24-hours <u>before</u> eruption until lesion becomes crusted. Lesions usually appear in different stages.

➤ Varicella (chicken pox):

Hx/PE: Myalgia, fever, pruritic painful lesions, and grouped dew drops on a "rose petal" that later show crusting. Palms and soles are spared. Adult onset is more severe and often complicated with pneumonia and encephalitis.

Note: Infected mothers with varicella need to be isolated from their babies. Infants <10 months have a 25% mortality rate.

➤ **Zoster (shingles)**:

Hx/PE: Dermatomal distribution that does <u>not</u> usually cross the midline, except in immunosuppressed patients. Local pain followed by grouped blisters on an erythematous base. Older patients may experience **post-herpetic neuralgia**.

Diagnosis: Clinical diagnosis or use Tzanck smear (multinucleated giant cells) for confirmation or PCR.

Treatment:

- <u>Toddlers</u>: require administration of acyclovir if age <10 months, immunosuppression, severe condition, or disseminated disease.

- <u>Children</u>: varicella is self-limiting but for patients aged >13 years then acyclovir is recommended.

- <u>Adults</u>: systemic or topical acyclovir can be used to minimize pain. Start treatment after clinical diagnosis.

- <u>Elderly</u>: do not need to isolate patients (if not disseminated) but should cover their lesions. Start treatment after clinical diagnosis.

- **Pregnancy**: can give vaccinations (<96 hours of exposure) <u>or</u> acyclovir (>98 hours of exposure) to pregnant mothers with varicella.

Note:

✓ Tzanck smear can detect both varicella-zoster and HSV.

✓ Post-herpetic neuralgia: can treat with desipramine (TCA), gabapentin, or pregabalin.

Molluscum contagiosum

Associated with *poxvirus (DNA virus)*, common in young children and AIDS patients. Spreads via physical contact and become tiny papules with "**central umbilication**." Lesions are also known as **water warts**.

Hx/PE:

➤ Children: lesions are on trunk, extremities, and face.

➤ Adults: Lesions are usually asymptomatica and around the genitalia and perineal region.

Diagnosis: Clinical diagnosis or excisional biopsy with Giemsa or Wright's stain (**molluscum bodies**).

Treatment:

- Self-limiting over months to years.

- Local destruction: curettage (scrape off), cryotherapy (liquid nitrogen, freezing), or trichloroacetic acid.

Verrucae (warts)

Caused by infection with *HPV strains* (130 different known types) which are transmission by direct contact. Warts are hyperproliferation of infected cells that tend to grow downwards into the skin with long intubation periods.

Hx/PE: Common in the hands, feet, genitals, and mucosa. Genital warts show classic "cauliflower-like" papules. Laryngeal warts more commonly seen in children, acquired from the mother's genital tract.

Diagnosis:

- Clinical diagnosis and acetowhitening (*confirmation*).

- Histological and cytological evaluation for malignancy, if lesions are present on the genitals.

Treatment: Curettage (scraping off), cryotherapy (freezing), salicylic acid, trichloroacetic acid, imiquimod, and podophyllin.

Dermatological bacterial infections

Acne vulgaris

Hormonal activation of sebaceous glands (comedo) or plugged

sebaceous follicle (*Propionibacterium acnes*).

Risk factors: comedos can be caused by genetics, anabolic steroids, menstrual cycle, puberty, GH, lithium, and corticosteroids. Can exacerbate cyclically with menstruation and androgenic stimulation. There is little correlation between acne and specific types of foods.

Hx/PE:

➤ **Comedo**: open comedo "black head" or closed comedo "white head."

➤ **Inflammatory**: sebaceous follicle plug, *Propionibacterium acnes*, large, and nodular.

➤ **Inflammatory cysts**: large and fluctuant pustules.

➤ **Epidermoid cysts**: on the eyebrows or behind the ears.

Diagnosis: Clinical diagnosis.

Treatment:

▪ *Mild inflammatory:* topical **benzoyl peroxide** 5% (*first line*), topical antibiotics, and/or topical retinoids (if topical antibiotics are not effective). Plus use water-based skin products verses oil-based products.

▪ *Moderate acne*: oral systemic antibiotics (minocycline or tetracycline) and/or *topical* retinoid.

▪ *Severe cystic acne and scarring*: oral isotretinoin, oral antibiotics (minocycline or clindamycin), and OCPs.

▪ *Increased androgens*: spironolactone (an anti-aldosterone diuretic that is used to treat acne in women owing to its anti-androgenic effects).

Note:

✓ As a rule of thumb, topical medications (benzoyl peroxide, antibiotics, and retinoids) are the *first-line medications* for mild to moderate disease.

✓ Oral medications (antibiotics and isotretinoin) are used in *severe* cases.

✓ Doxycycline has more photosensitivity effects than minocycline.

✓ If consideration of isotretinoin or tazarotene, need to ask about possible pregnancy and place on OCPs.

Side effects of isotretinoin:

- Increases levels of cholesterol and triglycerides, liver toxicity, **teratogenic** effects, and depression.
- Keep in mind that elevated triglycerides can cause pancreatitis; so avoid alcohol intake.
- Monthly hCG tests needed for refills, and two forms of birth control must be used, starting 1 month prior to treatment and 1 month after treatment (no exceptions).

Cellulitis

A bacterial infection that can effect various layer including the dermis, ubcutaneous layers, connective tissue and muscle. Common etiological factors are staphylococci and streptococci. Can develop into more serious infections such as necrotizing fasciitis or osteomyelitis.

Risk factors: IV drug use, trauma, venous stasis, and diabetes. If a patient uses black-tar heroin, infection with *clostridium* is likely.

Hx/PE: The erythemic borders are not generally sharply demarcated like in vasculitis. On physical examination, the skin is red, hot, swollen, and tender. Patients may also present with fever and chills.

Diagnosis:

- Always mark the area to monitor progression.
- Clinical diagnosis or can obtain wound culture if unsure of etiology.
- Blood culture if patient appears ill or has high fever.

Note: with cellulitis rule out osteomyelitis, DVT (if in lower extremity), and necrotizing fasciitis (NF).

Treatment:

- *Mild cellulitis*: oral antibiotics (cephalexin or dicloxacillin).
- *Severe cellulitis:* IV antibiotics (nafcillin or oxacillin) if systemic, involves the hands, feet, orbital regions, or the patient has comorbid disorders.
- If diabetic, then hospitalize and assess antibiotic sensitivities (vancomycin usually required).

Note: Local anesthetics often are not helpful since the local infections acid environment can neutralize the anesthetic.

Folliculitis

An inflammation of the hair follicle. Can be associated with *staphylococci* and *streptococci*. If history of hot tub use consider p*seudomonas*. Not present on palms or soles of hands and feet.

Etiology: staphylococcus, streptococcal, fungal, or mechanical (friction or shaving).

Hx/PE: Tiny pustule at the opening of the hair follicle.

➤ **Furuncle**: smaller collection of fluid.

➤ **Boils**: about 1 cm in size, tender, red papule, or fluctuant nodule.

➤ **Carbuncle**: several centimeters in size, tender, red papules that more commonly seen in diabetes or patients with immunosuppression.

Diagnosis: Clinical diagnosis or biopsy (rule out MRSA).

Treatment:

- *Mild*: topical antibiotics (**mupirocin** or **neomycin**).
- *Severe*: systemic oral antibiotics (**dicloxacillin**).
- *If abscess:* incision and drainage plus oral antibiotics.
- *Fungal infection*: oral fluconazole.

Note: In case of ingrown hairs, patients must avoid shaving as this can cause further irritation.

Impetigo

A bacterial infection caused by direct contact (highly contagious) and often presents with local lymphadenopathy. Infection to children are usually caused by group A streptococcus (*streptococcus pyogenes*) or staphylococcus (*staphylococcus aureus*).

> ➤ **Nonbullous type**: most common type. Causes pustules ("**honey-colored crusts on erythematous base**"); usually located by the nose or mouth.

> ➤ **Bullous type**: large painless <u>stable</u> blister that when busts will crust over with yellow fluid. Usually found in children on the extremities or trunk. Commonly caused by *S. aureus,* and can be complicated by acute streptococcal glomerulonephritis.

Diagnosis: Clinical diagnosis ("**honey crusted lesion**"), and confirm with culture (Gram stain).

Treatment:

- *Mild*: topical antibiotics (mupirocin).
- *Severe*: systemic antibiotics (nafcillin or oxacillin).

Note: Dicloxacillin can be an alternative.

Staphylococcal scaled skin syndrome (SSSS)

Causes damage in the epidermis by destroying desmosomes secondary to the release of *exotoxins*, released by staphylococcus aureus. Patients can become dehydrated and experience electrolyte imbalances.

Diagnosis: Clinical diagnosis (<u>positive</u> Nikolsky's sign) and positive Gram stain for staphylococcu.

Treatment:

- Antibiotics nafcillin and oxacillin (for MSSA) or vancomycin (for MRSA).
- Control: fluids, electrolytes, temperature, and infections.

Erythema multiforme (EM)

The direct cause is unknown but appears secondary to immune complex Ig's in the microvasculature of the skin (superficial layers). Cutaneous lesions with classic targetoid lesion appearance and commonly follow an infection or medication exposure. Can develop into toxic epidermal necrolysis TEN and Stevens-Johnson syndrome (SJS).

Risk factors: recurrent HSV, mycoplasma, coccidioidomycosis, and use of sulfas, NSAIDs, barbiturates, and penicillin.

Hx/PE: Can presents with arthralgia's and myalgia's and common on the palms and soles and less likely to occur on the mucous membrane. The lesions have a dusky "target appearance" and can develop into a blister.

Diagnosis: Clinical impression: target-like papules with an erythematous outer boarder, an inner pale ring, and a purple necrotic center. Rule out recurrent labial herpes, which is strongly associated.

Treatment:

- *In mild cases*, usually self-limiting; administer anti-pruritic (itching) and acyclovir (for recurrent herpes).

- *In severe cases,* treat in burn unit with high fluids and electrolyte replacement.

- Steroids are often not useful.

Stevens-Johnson syndrome (SJS)

Medical emergency

A type of toxic epidermal necrolysis, which causes cell death (necrosis) and destruction of the epidermis-dermis junction. Involves <10% of the skin with extensive mucosal and skin involvement. Appears to be an immune system activated response.

Risks: both TEN and SJS can be caused by use of sulfonamides, NSAIDs, barbiturates, penicillin, and anti-seizure medications.

Hx/PE: Usually presents with flu-like symptoms (fever, fatigue, and sore throat). Then later, ulcers start to appear on mucous membranes and skin. Skin tenderness and often +Nikolsky's sign.

Diagnosis: CBC, electrolytes, ESR, urinalysis, BUN/Cr ratio, and skin biopsy (degeneration of the basal layer of the epidermis. Some eosinophils and possible subepidermal blisters.

Treatment:

- *First step* is to discard offending agents.
- Treat similar to burn patient: IV fluids, electrolyte replacement, thermoregulation, and infection control.
- Treatment is controversial with corticosteroids and debridement.

Toxic epidermal necrolysis (TEN)

Medical emergency

Usually caused by a reaction to a medication, which causes an immune response and the separation of the epidermis from the dermis, secondary to keratinocyte destruction. Involves >30% of the skin leading to necrosis of the full epidermis. SJS/TEN can overlap and considered when between 10%-30% of body is involved. TEN has a high mortality rate and can lead to sepsis.

Hx/PE: Usually presents with flu-like symptoms and then later with skin tenderness, redness, necrosis, and +Nikolsky's sign.

Diagnosis:

- Order: CBC, ESR, urinalysis, LFTs, BUN/Cr ratio, and electrolyte panel.
- Blood culture (rule out sepsis), plain radiography (to determine extent), and/or CT scan (extent)
- *Most accurate:* biopsy of full-thickness skin (eosinophilic epidermal necrosis).

Treatment:

- *First step* is to remove offending agents.
- Treatment in the burn unit or ICU: IV fluids, electrolyte replacement, thermoregulation, infection control.
- Controversial treatment with corticosteroids and debridement.

Necrotizing fasciitis (NF)

Medical emergency

Deep infection along the fascial plane and within the subcutaneous tissues. Often caused by *S. pyogenes* or *Clostridium perfringens* (gas production) which can progresse rapidly and become fatal. Often occurs after trauma or surgery.

Hx/PE: Sudden onset of severe pain and swelling at the site of trauma or surgery. Erythema quickly spreads within hours to days. These dusky or purplish lesions quickly lead to necrosis of the deep fascia.

Diagnosis:

- Medical emergency (start IV Zosyn, clindamycin, and vancomycin before work-up).
- *Best initial test*: radiography or CT scan (air in tissue).
- Order: CBC, electrolytes, urinalysis, BUN/Cr ratio, and CPK level tests.
- *Most accurate*: biopsy culture (edge of tissue; test is *diagnostic*).

Note: Always mark lesion perimeters to monitor progression.

Treatment:

- IV antibiotics (<u>cannot</u> be used alone, as surgical debridement is required).
- Start with Zosyn, clindamycin, and vancomycin until sensitivities are available.
  - If group A streptococcus: penicillin G and clindamycin.
  - If anaerobic infections: metronidazole or cephalosporin.
- Emergent surgical debridement (absolutely required for treatment).
- Volume status is important for monitoring purposes.

Seborrheic dermatitis

An inflammatory skin disorder where the direct cause is unknown but appears to have some involvement with *Pityrosporum ovale (malassezia furfur)*. There is also an association with Parkinson's disease, HIV, and epilepsy.

Hx/PE: Characterized by erythematous and scaling plaques that typically affects the scalp (dandruff), ears, face, eyebrows, and central chest.

Diagnosis: Clinical diagnosis and need to rule out HIV in newly diagnosed patients.

Treatment: Ketoconazole shampoo and artificial UV radiation.

Note: HIV testing always requires consent.

Ludwig's angina

Can cause a life-threatening cellulitis or connective tissue infection of the submaxillary or sublingual areas of the mouth, usually caused by an infected tooth. Can cause asphyxiation.

Hx/PE: Dysphagia, drooling, fever, erythemia, and warm mouth.

Diagnosis: History and physical examination with clinical findings after a dental procedure.

Treatment:

- Monitor respiratory and airway status.
- Antibiotics of choice are penicillin-based antibiotics; consult dentistry for incision and drainage.

Erythrasma

A skin disease that is caused by *Corynebacterium*.

Hx/PE: Brownish-red scaly patches that involves major skin folds and is common in diabetes.

Diagnosis: **Wood's light** (fluoresce a "coral–red" color).

Treatment: Oral erythromycin.

Gangrene

Necrosis of the body tissue most commonly caused by decreased blood supply. Commonly seen in diabetics and smokers.

Types:

➤ **Dry gangrene**: insufficient blood flow to tissues (example;

atherosclerosis).

- **Wet gangrene**: bacterial infection usually caused by skin flora; which also disrupts blood flow.

- **Gas gangrene**: (**Medical emergency**) *C. perfringens* (common) infection leads to gas production and separates healthy skin tissue. The skin first turns pale and later dark red. Common with recent injury or surgery.

Diagnosis: Clinical diagnosis and biopsy (Gram stain), if needed.

Treatment:

- *Dry gangrene:* antibiotics are not useful, as dry gangrene is not caused by infection.
  - For dry gangrene need to consider revascularization.
- *Wet gangrene:* antibiotics and surgical debridement.
- *Gas gangrene*: emergency surgery, hyperbaric oxygen, antibiotics, and surgical debridement.

Note: Consider amputation if aggressive management is ineffective.

Pilonidal cysts

Abscess in the sacrococcygeal region that occurs at the top of the natal cleft. Repetitive trauma to the region plays an etiological role. Thought to start as a folliculitis that develops into an abscess.

Hx/PE: Abscess on the natal cleft and on physical examination, observe a cluctuant, tender, warm, indurated, and a purulent drainage.

Diagnosis: Clinical diagnosis but need to rule rule out perirectal and anal abscess.

Treatment:

- Incision and drainage and allow the abscess to heal with secondary intention Ensure good local hygiene, and shave the area.
- Antibiotics, if needed (reserved for immunocompromised, large [>5cm], or systemic infections).

Dermatological fungal infections

Candidiasis

Most commonly caused by *C. albicans* (fungus) which tends to affect moist areas such as, under the breasts, diaper area, groin, axilla, vagina, and feet.

Risk factors: Use of antibiotics, steroids, inhaled steroids, immuno-suppression, recent birth, obesity, and diabetes.

Hx/PE:

➤ **Oral candidiasis**: white painless plaques that are easy to wipe off.

  • Rule out HIV infection, unless there is an obvious risk factor.

➤ **Superficial candidiasis**: pink circular erythematous macules.

Diagnosis:

- Clinical diagnosis.
- *Best initial test*: scraping or swabbing the affected area and use microscopic evaluation with 10% KOH solution (visualize pseudohyphae or budding yeast).
- *Most accurate test*: fungus culture.

Note: The KOH dissolves the cell membrane but leaves the candida cells intact.

Treatment:

- *Oral candida*: nystatin swish and swallow or oral fluconazole.
- *Superficial*: topical anti-fungal medication and keep skin dry.
- *Diaper rash* (rash usually includes skin folds): Topical nystatin.
- *Severe cases*: amphotericin B.

Tinea versicolor

A type of fungus known as *pityriasis versicolor* (normal flora of the skin) and more commonly found in humid conditions and patients with oily skin.

Hx/PE: Small, scaly patches of varying colors found on the chest and back.

> - <u>Hypopigmentation</u>: caused by interference in melanin production.

> - <u>Hyperpigmentation</u>: caused by thickened scales.

Diagnosis:

- Clinical diagnosis or KOH test ("**spaghetti and meatball**" pattern of hyphae and spores).
- Usually skin culture or biopsy are not needed.

Treatment: Treatment of choice is <u>topical</u> antifungal therapy (selenium disulfide, ketoconazole shampoos, or terbinafine).

Dermatophyte infections

More commonly found in tissues with high levels of *keratin* (skin, nail, and hair).

> - **Tinea corporis** (body): scaly pruritic lesions with a sharp irregular border often with central clearing.

> - **Tinea pedis** (foot): also known as athlete's foot. interdigital scaling (between toes) and scaly skin on the soles of the feet.

> - **Tinea cruris** (jock itch): located in the groin area and typically sparing the scrotum.

> - **Tinea capitis** (scalp): scaly scalp eruptions, similar to seborrheic dermatitis.

Diagnosis: Clinical diagnosis or KOH test (shows hyphae or spores).

Treatment:

- *Mild infection*: use topical antifungals.
- *Severe infection*: use systemic antifungals.
- Tinea capitis and onychomycosis require oral antifungals,

administer **terbinafine** ([first-line treatment] can cause liver toxic) or itraconazole.

Note: Always remember to educate patients about keeping susceptible areas dry.

Dermatological parasitic infections

Enterobius vermicularis (pinworm)

A parasitic worm commonly found in the intestinal tract. The female parasite lays eggs at night in the outer anal area, which causes perianal irritation and pruritus in the mornings.

Hx/PE: Commonly causes pruritus of the anal and pelvic area.

Diagnosis: Scotch tape test on the perianal area (can visualize eggs and larvae).

Treatment: **Oral mebendazole** or **albendazole**.

Louse (lice)

Lice live off blood and skin tissue and spread with contact or by sharing garments or bedclothes.

Types of human louse: head louse, body louse, and pubic louse (crabs).

Hx/PE: More common in crowded environments and epidemic areas. Patients with severe pruritus.

- ➤ Body louse: crowded living or unhygienic conditions.
- ➤ Head louse: common in elementary classrooms.
- ➤ Pubic louse: have anticoagulant in the saliva (blue bites).

Diagnosis: Lice are visible (use tweezers [mechanically remove] and magnifying glass [help visualize]).

Treatment:

- <u>Head, body, and pubic lice</u>: topical permethrin and mechanical removal.
- Need to question family members about similar symptoms and educate on washing clothes, bedding, and body hygiene.

Note: Permethrin can be purchased over the counter.

Scabies

Sarcoptes scabiei is an arthropod, in which females lays eggs in the *stratum corneum* (creating "vein-like channels" under skin).

Hx/PE: Extreme pruritus (histamine release) with symptoms usually in several family members that worsen at night or after a hot shower. Common in the axillae, webs of fingers and toes, genitals, and breast.

Diagnosis: Microscopic examination (mite tracks).

Treatment: 5% topical permethrin from the neck down (1–2 applications) plus treat contacts.

Vascular dermatology

Senile purpura

Senile purpura is a benign condition seen more commonly in elderly patients and characterized by recurrent formation of blue/purple ecchymosis. Common after minor trauma and patients who are on topical steroids (which things the skin) and blood thinners.

Hx/PE: Irregular shaped purple-blue macules.

Diagnosis: Clinical diagnosis; no further work-up needed.

Treatment:

- Benign and self-limiting.

- Sun protection (long-sleeve shirts, sunscreen, and avoiding afternoon sun).

Bacillary angiomatosis

A form of angiomatosis that is associated with *bartonella* bacteria. Common in HIV-infected patients.

Hx/PE: "Bright red firm nodules."

Diagnosis: Clinical diagnosis and should rule out HIV.

Treatment: Can be fatal. Treatment with erythromycin or doxycycline.

Strawberry hemangiomas

Benign vascular involvement of the *endothelial* cells that line the blood vessels. Usually appear in the first weeks of live and generally regress by the age of 8 years. In some cases the hemangiomas do not regress.

Diagnosis: Clinical diagnosis.

Treatment: Steroids and β-blockers.

Cherry hemangiomas

Also known as **senile hemangiomas,** which can increase in numbers with age. They are benign vascular tumors seen in adults due to an abnormal growth of blood vessels (capillaries).

Hx/PE: Appear as red dome-shaped papules. Do not regress spontaneously and do not usually require treatment.

Diagnosis: Clinical diagnosis.

Treatment: On rare occasions, consider cryosurgery or electrosurgery.

Stasis dermatitis

Stasis dermatitis

Persistent inflammation of the skin due to insufficient venous return. Commonly related to venous insufficiency and can progress to cellulitis. Usually presents bilaterally with hyperpigmentation and scaling of the overlying skin.

Diagnosis: Clinical diagnosis; assess circulation function and signs of heart failure.

Treatment:

- Exercise and movement with elevation of lower extremities while resting.
- Compression stockings.
- Topical corticosteroids for alleviating pruritus and scaling.

Decubitus ulcers

Caused by continuous pressure, restricted microcirculation, confinement to the bed, and lack of mobility. Can develop ischemic necrosis of tissues.

Hx/PE:

- Stage 1: redness, irritation, and soreness.
- Stage 2: ulcerations of epidermis, dermis, or both.
- Stage 3: ulcerations of full thickness of subcutaneous tissue that extends to but not through the underlying fascia.
- Stage 4: ulcers full thickness loss with extensive tissue loss that can damage, muscle, tendons, and bone.

Diagnosis: Clinical appearance.

Treatment:

- Physical therapy, special beds, and wound care.
- Grade 3 and 4, pack ulcers with saline-moist gauze to preserve moisture.
- Surgical debridement and antibiotics (in severe cases).

Dermatology benign tumors

Acrochordons (skin tags)

More commonly seen in diabetics and obese patients. <u>Benign</u> light brown pedunculated lesions common in the neck, axilla, and groin area.

Diagnosis: Clinical diagnosis.

Treatment: For cosmetic reasons use surgical excision or liquid nitrogen (freeze).

Seborrheic keratosis

A benign skin tumor of unknown etiology.

Hx/PE: Hyperpigmented lesions, waxy "stuck on" appearance, and "greasy" or horned pseudocysts.

Diagnosis: Clinical diagnosis or skin biopsy (basaloid epidermal cells and "horn pseudocysts").

Treatment:

- No treatment required (benign).
- For symptomatic or cosmetic reasons: use liquid nitrogen (cryotherapy) or curettage.

Dermatological skin cancers

Actinic keratosis

Precursor to squamous cell carcinoma (SCC) in about 20% of the cases. Common in fair-skinned patients and elderly population with chronic sun exposure.

Hx/PE: More commonly seen in sun-exposed areas such as, hands, scalp, ears, face, upper chest, and forearms. Lesions can appear rough with keratotic papules that can become thick and crusted.

Diagnosis:

- Clinical diagnosis.
- Biopsy is seldom necessary (if carcinoma suspected, rapidly growing, thick, bleeding, or >1cm in diameter; then perform biopsy).
    - Common biopsy methods are shave biopsy and punch biopsy.

Treatment: Options: cryosurgery (local low temperature), surgical excision, topical retinoic acid derivatives, topical 5-FU cream, or topical imiquimod.

Squamous cell carcinoma (SCC)

SCC is an epithelial cancer that develops more commonly in sun-exposed areas. Common in fair-skinned patients and elderly patients. Usually benign with low risk of metastasis (about 3–7%).

Risk factors: UV light, chemicals, radiation, arsenic, tobacco smoking, chronic draining of infected sinuses, and actinic keratosis.

Diagnosis: Clinical diagnosis and biopsy (full thickness at the edge of the mass). Histological findings intraepidermal atypical "keratinocytes."

Treatment:

- Benign: surgical excision (**Mohs surgery**).
- Malignant: excision followed by radiation and/or chemotherapy.
- Others: imiquimod.

Basal cell carcinoma (BCC)

Most common malignant skin tumor, more likely found on sun exposed areas with a 95% cure rate.

Risk factors: UV light, sun exposure, arsenic exposure (non-sun exposed areas), or inherited basal cell nevus syndrome.

Diagnosis:

- Clinical diagnosis ("pearly" and flesh-colored papule).
- Shave biopsy or punch biopsy (shows islands of epithelium resembling the basal layer of the epidermis.).

Treatment: Surgical excision, deep cryotherapy, superficial radiation, and Mohs surgery.

Prevention: avoid outdoor activities during high noon and wear protective clothing.

Melanoma

Most common life-threatening dermatologic disease, mainly because of unpredictable growth and metastasis. Begins in the epidermal basal layer where the melanocytes are found. Usually flat in the initial stages with horizontal growth. Becomes dangerous with vertical growth and dermal invasion.

Risk factors: highly associated with UV radiation exposure. Short intense burst of sun exposure, congenital melanocytic nevi, and familial atypical mole (FAM-M syndrome).

Hx/PE: Lesions are more concerning when "ABCD": Asymmetry, borders irregular, color change, diameter change or deep growth. Unpredictable timeframe of metastasis and migrates to random places.

- ➤ **Superficial spread** (*most common* [70%]): prolonged horizontal growth phase.
- ➤ **Lentigo maligna**: arises from a lentigo; sun-damaged skin areas; common among the elderly; good prognosis.
- ➤ **Nodular** (15%): rapid vertical growth. Can present with ulceration and hemorrhage.
- ➤ **Acral lentiginous**: originates in the hands and feet (high morality).
- ➤ **Melanoma in situ**: originates in the dermis; 100% cure rate.

Diagnosis:

- Early detection is critical.
- Pruritus can be an early sign of malignancy.

- Requires <u>excisional biopsy:</u> staging based on **Breslow's classification** (thickness) <u>or</u> **Clark's classification**, or **TNM** (tumor size, # nodes, and metastasis).

- Familial melanoma syndrome is associated with cyclin-dependent kinase inhibitor 2A (CKDN2A) tumor suppressor gene.

Treatment:

- *First step* is aggressive excisional biopsy with wide margins (≥1cm).

    - Node dissection is used for staging.

- If depth is <1.0mm, then perform 1cm margin excision and no further test.

- If depth is >1.0mm, then perform lymph node biopsy.

- Radiation and chemotherapy can be used but are not usually successful.

Kaposi's sarcoma

A vascular proliferative disease. Most commonly associated with malignancy in HIV patients. Also ssociated with HHV-8, DM, advanced age, and HIV with CD4 <100 (more aggressive).

Hx/PE: Multicentric purplish vascular macules on the lower extremities.

Diagnosis: Clinical diagnosis or biopsy (spinal cells, elongated tumor cells, with positive HHV-8 staining).

Treatment: Technically palliative, HAART medications, cryotherapy, radiation, and systemic chemotherapy (IFN-α).

Note: Surgery is not recommended.

Cosmetic dermatology

➤ Wrinkles are deeper and higher in numbers in cigarette smokers than in non-smokers.

➤ Tretinoin (all-trans-retinoic acid) has been approved by the FDA for fine wrinkles and mottled hyperpigmentation.

➤ Use protective clothing for preventing skin exposure to the sun, which helps prevent sun damage.

➤ Laser tattoo removal can lead to scarring and skin discoloration.

➤ The most reasonable recommendations for sun protection is wearing protective clothing and sunscreen (30 minutes before sun exposure). Avoiding intense sun exposure from 10 am–4 pm, is recommended but not always reasonable.

Index

A

acanthosis nigricans 6
acne vulgaris 16
acrochordons 31
actinic keratosis 32
albendazole 28
anti-desmoglein antibodies 10
anti-melanocyte 11
arthus reaction 4
atopic dermatitis 2

B

bacillary angiomatosis 29
basal cell carcinoma 33
Behcet's syndrome 14
benzoyl peroxide 17
boils 19
Breslow's classification 34
bullous pemphigoid 10

C

candidiasis 25
carbuncle 19
celiac disease 13
cellulitis 18
cherry hemangiomas 30
chicken pox 14
Clark's classification 34
comedo 17
contact dermatitis 3

D

decubitus ulcers 31
dermatitis herpetiformis 13
desmoglein 9
diaper rash 26
dicloxacillin 19
disseminated herpes zoster 14

E

eczema 2
enterobius vermicularis 28
epidermoid cysts 17
erythema multiforme 20
erythrasma 24

F

familial melanoma syndrome 34
FAM-M syndrome 34
fixed drug eruption 8
folliculitis 19
furuncle 19

G

gangrene 24
gas gangrene: 24

H

hemangiomas 30
herpes simplex virus 13
H&E staining 10
hives 8
hypersensitivity reactions 3, 4

I

impetigo 19
inflammatory cysts 17

K

Kaposi's sarcoma 35
keloids 11
Koebner's phenomena 12
Koebner's phenomenon 6

L

laryngeal warts 16
lentigo 34

Index, con't.